Vocal Abuse
Reduction Program

Vocal Abuse Reduction Program

Thomas S. Johnson, PhD

Department of Communicative Disorders
Utah State University
Logan, Utah

pro·ed

8700 Shoal Creek Boulevard
Austin, Texas 78757

Printed in the United States of America

Library of Congress Cataloging-in-Publication Data

Johnson, Thomas, 1941–
    Vocal abuse reduction program / Thomas S. Johnson.
      p.   cm.
    Includes bibliographical references and index.
    ISBN 0-89079-314-X
    1. Voice disorders—Treatment.   2. Voice disorders—Patients–
  Rehabilitation. I. Title.
RF510.J64   1991
616.85'505—dc20   90-20892
                                        CIP

pro·ed
8700 Shoal Creek Boulevard
Austin, Texas 78757

2   3   4   5   6   7   8   9   10   97   96   95   94   93

TABLE OF CONTENTS

PREFACE

The VARP manual is intended to be a programmatic manual for the clinician in speech-language pathology. Its contents have been organized for easy understanding and efficient use. This data-based program, if used properly, will facilitate the remediation of hyperfunctional voice problems. The first chapter of the manual describes the program and its components. Chapter 2 provides a variety of clinical forms and materials for use with the program. Chapter 3 contains the program outlines that may be used by the clinician to plan specific clinical activities.

Appendix A provides materials for use in VARP workshops or other in-service training activities. These have been included to facilitate formal training workshops for hyperfunctional voice disorders, although the manual is intended to be generally self-instructional.

A microcomputer program is also available from College-Hill Press, which provides microcomputer controlled training in VARP procedures as well as data storage and retrieval capability for clinical use. These materials are valuable adjuncts to the basic VARP procedures outlined in this manual.

ACKNOWLEDGMENTS

I am grateful to many individuals for the work that has been done in the development of this program as well as in the other areas of voice research, at Utah State University. I particularly would like to acknowledge those individuals who have completed thesis research projects under my direction, as they contributed greatly to the development of this and other voice management programs. Included in these efforts were Jolene C. Hunsaker, Madelyn L. Parrish, Linda R. Beste, Deenaz Coachbuilder, Gretchen Greiner, Roxann Rothwell, Ginger L. Pierce, Melody S. Beck, Cheri F. Cornaby, Susan Williams, Connie Thompson, Sonny Vance, Terry Taylor, Joanne Inglis, Jean Ernstrom, Dee R. Child, and Kim Williams. These individuals performed the research and clinical work utilizing these experimental clinical procedures under pressure of direct observation and supervision. Thanks must also go to the beautiful children who participated in our clinical experiment for their outstanding efforts in responding to the clinicians and the program assignments. To Don, Gordon, Craig, Brent, Troy, Melanie, and all the other hyperfunctional voice children I express my thanks. Their parents must also be included as unsung heroes for their determination and cooperation during the experimental development of the clinical program.

Furthermore, I am grateful for the continual assistance and support received from the Department of Communicative Disorders, particularly from Jay R. Jensen, Jaclyn Littledike, and Carol Strong, and from the College of Education at Utah State University to work on research in voice disorders. I have also appreciated the opportunities to share data and information with individuals and groups throughout the country. Their feedback, enthusiasm and acceptance provided important social reinforcers as well as crucial suggestions for the betterment of the VARP procedures. A special note of appreciation must go to the Montana State Office of the Superintendent of Public Instruction for funding the Montana VARP field project and especially to Douglas Wing, the project director, Shirley DeVoe, Marilyn Pearson, and the clinicians of that state who participated in that significant effort. Wing's challenge to give VARP a fair chance in the public schools was an important turning point in the continued progress of this program. More recently Dee Child has provided much valuable assistance in the transfer of this Program to a microcomputer format. His enthusiasm and devotion to quality has kept my motivation for this project high.

Finally, I am indebted to the support of my choice family who share me in far too many extrafamilial activities. This effort is dedicated with love and appreciation to them.

Chapter 1

The Vocal Abuse Reduction Program

PURPOSE AND BACKGROUND

The purpose of this clinical program is to pinpoint vocal abuse behaviors and to reduce them systematically in certain specific high frequency situations. The reduction of vocal abuse behavior has been demonstrated to reduce the size or eliminate the presence of vocal nodules, polyps, contact ulcers, or other forms of laryngeal pathology resulting from vocal abuse-misuse. This reduction facilitates normal voice quality.

Early in 1969, work was begun in the use of self-counting or monitoring procedures by clients with vocal nodules (Johnson, 1971). This procedure appeared to have an immediate but temporary effect in improving vocal quality. A 10 year old male client was asked as part of his therapy to self-count his yelling behavior during the course of his communicating day. His daily behavior record showed a large deceleration in yelling for about three weeks before he stopped counting.

Further research and development resulted in a clinical treatment program (Johnson and Parrish, 1972) that has been successful in reducing hyperfunctional behaviors related to the voice, particularly in the remediation of vocal nodules. The vocal abuse reduction program (VARP) is data based, and the success rate in clinical settings has been very high (more than 95 per cent). Some early reports indicated basic problems with this approach in the public school setting (Gordon, 1971), and so a special form of the program was designed and used in a pilot research study (Beck, 1974) aimed at investigating whether the modified program could be used efficiently in public school speech programs. The results of that study indicated that the program lost its efficiency by about half in its application to the public school situation. Subsequently, the VARP was field tested on a wide scale in public school regions in the state of Montana with considerable success (Wing, Johnson, DeVoe, and Pearson, 1975). The results of that project indicated that the VARP program was effective in public school settings with proper administration and efficient utilization of professional resources. Hence, the VARP may be considered a universally applicable program for voice problems resulting from abuse-misuse of the vocal mechanism. When administered properly, it is effective both in the highly controlled clinic situation and in public school speech and hearing programs.

The vocal abuse reduction program is a clinical management program that pinpoints vocal abuse behaviors for each client with vocal abuse behaviors that have resulted in laryngeal pathologies of various types such as nodules, polyps, contact ulcers, thickened vocal records, and so forth. The program then systematically reduces the pinpointed vocal abuse behaviors in specific high probability situations or time periods, and finally reduces the size or eliminates laryngeal pathology (of abuse-misuse etiology) and makes possible the establishment of normal vocal quality.

DEVELOPMENT

The program components have been developed through research studies and clinical experience and have been placed in the program to combat specific clinical problems which arose in the therapeutic process. The rationale for each component will be discussed below, but it should be stated that close adherence to the outlined program procedures is of paramount importance. There appear to be no shortcuts available in the efficient management of vocal abuse. Therefore, *all* components of the VARP have been included because they have been found to be necessary. Any deviation from the outlined procedures will probably cause the clinician to discover the same blind alleys and log-jams that have already been encountered in the development of the program. VARP has been demonstrated to work; a modification of VARP may not. Several years of problem solving with VARP users have demonstrated that problems running VARP are almost always related to improper program administration.

The VARP has undergone 12 years of formative development. The initial two years were chiefly experimental-clinical attempts to utilize self-monitoring as a tool in voice therapy. The subsequent years were a series of clinical application studies which resulted in refinements, additions, and modifications of the program concept. Several single subject studies have been completed using the program, and the 1972 and 1976 versions of the program have been used in many clinic settings including Utah State University, Primary Children's Medical Center in Salt Lake City, the Easter Seal Rehabilitation Center in Bridgeport, Connecticut, and in other settings in Pennsylvania, Iowa, Arizona, Oregon, Montana, Vermont, and California. Unsolicited reports of its successful application have been frequent. Problems with the program have also been reported to the author, and either appropriate changes have been implemented or problem solving has shown incorrect implementation of the program procedures (see *Branching–Clinical Alternatives*). The clinical studies completed at Utah State University under close scrutiny of the author have demonstrated a success rate of more than 95 per cent with the 1972, 1974, and the 1976 editions in the clinical setting. The development of the program has gone on concurrently with clinical research efforts in other areas of voice disorders (Johnson, 1974, 1985).

Specific research data may be found in Beck (1974), Hunsaker (1970), Johnson (1971, 1985), Johnson and Parrish (1972), Johnson and Wing (1976; in preparation), Parrish (1972), and Wing et al. (1975), as well as in unpublished data at Utah State University. The table found on page 66 provides general success data on the programs during the development of the VARP. A recently published microcomputer program (Johnson and Child, 1984) provides complete training and data collection, retrieval, and storage capability for clinicians. The training program can stand as an in-service training experience on the VARP with Continuing Education Unit (CEU) credit available from Utah State University.

PROGRAM COMPONENTS

Pinpointing. It is important to pinpoint the form of vocal abuse behavior that occurs most frequently with the individual child in order to eliminate it. The behavior must be specified in behavioral form, that is, it must be countable and observable. Such vocal abuse behaviors may include loud talks and yells, throat clearing, coughing, motor noises, strained vocalization, and so forth. These abuse behaviors will vary from individual to individual and care must be taken to pinpoint accurately those abuse behaviors that are clinically operative in each individual. An example of this importance of this pinpointing process occurred during a pilot study conducted in connection with the development of the program. The pinpointed behavior of loud talks and yells in a 10 year old boy was reduced to two abuses per day after several weeks. The nodules reduced some, but were not entirely eliminated. Further investigation of the boy's behavior revealed that he rode his bicycle regularly to school and would pretend that he was on a motorcycle. To change the gears he made loud "motor noises" with his voice. In this case, important vocal abuse behavior had not been accurately pinpointed. Loud talks and yells were not the sole source of the vocal abuse behavior which this child had in his daily living pattern. In addition, vocal misuse behaviors such as inadequate breath control may also be important to observe and pinpoint. Respiratory, resonatory, and phonatory behaviors must be considered as each has the potential for contributing to a hyperfunctional voice problem.

Self-Counting. Self-monitoring of behavior has been shown to be an effective means of developing control of behavior (Edwards and Powers, 1973; Foster, 1974; Lindsley, 1968; Miller, 1980). This technology utilizes self-monitored continuous or programmed tracking of personal behaviors. Self-monitoring apparently brings those behaviors to a conscious level and also provides a form of consequent event following the behavior in the form of tallying on a counter or other type of record whenever the behavior occurs. This record can then be monitored over a period of days, weeks, months, or years utilizing a daily behavior chart. Changes in the frequency of the behavior can then be seen from day to day over the time period the record is kept. Various types of intervention strategies can also be programmed into the process which can assist in the deceleration or acceleration of specific behaviors as desired. The VARP uses self-counting of vocal abuse behaviors by the individual in an effort to either reduce or eliminate those behaviors and thus improve laryngeal efficiency and facilitate the healing of laryngeal tissues. Traditionally, friends, teachers, clinicians, and parents were given the major responsibility of tracking vocal abuse behavior. These individuals were effective as long as they were with the child and as long as they remembered to monitor the child's behavior; however, motivation in these individuals was difficult to maintain and highly variable monitoring resulted. Self-counting by the individual provides a means for more consistent, accurate, and complete data collection as well as a means for developing behavioral control more quickly in the natural environment.

Initially, concern was expressed about the reliability of self-monitoring; however, in the early studies it was found that individuals who counted and collected their own data were reliable as their reports agreed with those of other observers in specific situations. In addition, it was found that they were honest in their reports and little if any problem has been found with falsified or "dry-lab" data. It also was found that the procedure worked—with the resulting decrease of vocal abuse behavior, laryngeal pathologies were eliminated! Thus, the early concern about reliability of the data was considered secondary to the fact of remediation, which was objectively observed. Precise counting of abuse behavior is not as important as the overall awareness and behavioral set regarding such behavior.

Parents, teachers, or other individuals in the environment can be used intermittently as occasional program aids as a reminder stimulus in the environment and perhaps as an accuracy check of the individual's counting. Self-counting has the additional advantage of introducing behavioral stimulus control into the client's environment. The use of a wrist counter may be likened to using a string tied around the finger as a reminder stimulus. As the program progresses the individual is counting and bringing under control his vocal abuse behaviors during increasingly greater portions of his communicative day. By the end of the program, the individual is tracking those behaviors during the entire day. This programmed monitoring aids in the generalization of behavioral control of vocal abuse behavior and facilitates carry-over.

Wrist Counters. The wrist counter is a functional addition to the tools of the speech clinician. Originally, wrist counters were developed for accurately recording golf scores. A modified version has been implemented to assist in the monitoring of behavior particularly in self-control studies. In the VARP, the wrist counter is used as a means for tallying the number of vocal abuse behaviors emitted and as an environmental stimulus to remind the individual on the program about his vocal usage. Because it is strapped to the wrist, it travels with the individual to all parts of his environment and is not easily ignored nor lost. In addition, it has been observed to have a novelty effect (as something new, different, and unique) with both adults and children and therefore may have some social reinforcing properties. If necessary, the counter may be made even more socially reinforcing by using an attractive fashionable band. This can assist in "motivation," particularly for children, and enhances the desirability of wearing the counter. The individual is instructed to wear the counter only during the time periods he is assigned to count for the program. Proper utilization in this regard can assure its continued effectiveness as a reminder stimulus in the environment in which the client is to be aware of vocal abuse behavior and in situations which have a high probability for such abuse behavior to occur. If initially it is worn continually, it may lose its reminder stimulus value. Hence, the wearing of the counter is carefully scheduled into the therapy program by the clinician.

High Probability Time Periods. The effectiveness of the VARP depends on the effectiveness of stimulus control techniques bringing vocal abuse behavior under control in a sequence of specific situations or periods of time. Therefore, the clinician must obtain an important body of information about each individual's environmental life pattern. This consists of finding out which situations in the individual's environment have a high probability for evoking vocal abuse behaviors.

Usually, this analysis results in a relatively small number of situations or times which then may be systematically sequenced for control within the VARP procedure. Clinical experience suggests that these situations will number from four to six in each individual. Bringing each of these situations under control is the central focus of the VARP.

In the early stages of program development, individuals in the program were required to count all vocal abuses during the entire day beginning with the first day of therapy. This procedure was temporarily successful, but cessation of self-counting behavior was noted after a couple of weeks. It was suggested that this cessation was due to either a loss of the novelty effect of the procedure or a lack of other motivational maintenance of the counting. As a result the VARP in its present form requires counting only one short period of time initially and then progresses to increased counting of the additional high probability time periods. Situational time periods, such as recesses, lunch periods, and various activity times, are effective because they are not only short, but also act as environmental reminder stimuli for counting. As the vocal abuse behavior is brought under control in each situation, a new situation is added thereby providing additional time for the individual to monitor. This procedure is repeated until all of the high probability situations or times are being monitored and the vocal abuse behavior is under control. When this point is reached, the individual can then be assigned to monitor his vocal behavior during the entire communicative day. If the behavior is not brought under control in a specific situation, then that situation may have to be worked on intensively by involving others in the environment, implementing a contingency management program, breaking the time period into smaller periods, or other appropriate "branching" techniques. Criterion levels have been determined for moving from situation to situation. These criterion levels are discussed in the general format instructions. Rigid adherence to the criterion levels is not necessary, but they do serve as a guide to progression through the program.

Daily Behavior Charting. The VARP is most effective for both the client and clinician if the standard Daily Behavior Chart (Behavior Research Company, Box 3351, Kansas City, KS 66103) is used. This standardized chart has many advantages for use with this program, such as the capability to demonstrate visually through the use of "behavioral floors" the client's progression during the time being monitored (Fig. 1). In addition, standard acceleration and accuracy data are helpful for the clinician in summarizing data and in providing descriptive material in reports, letters, presentations, and so forth. Also, the chart can be used for one half of a school year and data can be kept on a daily basis including weekends. The use of the standard Daily Behavior Chart is described in detail in Koorland and Martin (1975), Kunzelmann, Cohen, Hulten, Martin, and Mingo (1970), White and Having (1980), and is described with relevance to speech-language pathology by Diedrich (1974) and Mowrer (1982). Other charts may be used with the program, but it is strongly felt that efficiency and total program tracking can be best achieved through the use of the Daily Behavior Chart. Descriptions of its use in conjunction with this program may be found in Beck (1974), Johnson and Wing (1976), Parrish (1972), Thompson (1976), and in the appended workshop materials (Appendix A).

In general, the charting for the VARP should be done by the clinician from the data supplied by the individual being seen for therapy. The program includes provisions for the charting to be done during each weekly session and the chart should be made available for the client to see. In some cases, it may be desirable to allow the client to do the actual charting or to keep a chart for himself; however, a duplicate should be kept by the clinician. Care must also be taken during review of the chart—there should be no suggestion that the data must go in a specific direction (up or down) which might provoke doctoring of actual data (see also *Reinforcements*).

Home Telephone Calls. Another extension or generalization strategy used in the VARP is the use of home telephone calls. These calls are carefully programmed into the therapy sequence initially to provide environmental reminder stimuli as well as to suggest to the client and others in his environment (parents, for example) of the importance of the program and the interest of the clinician in seeing that the program is effective. If the individual knows he or she will receive a telephone call at night asking for the day's data, he or she will be encouraged to remember to count abusive behavior and to be ready to report. The home calls also supply stimuli to parents and others to remind the individual to count his or her abusive behaviors. Additionally, the call is a good time to correct any problems that the individual may have in connection with the program and problem solving can thus take place immediately. As the program progresses and the individual is satisfactorily collecting data, the calls may be faded out. They are, however, a critical and necessary part of the VARP. Attempts to leave home telephone calls out of the program have failed. Proper administration of the VARP requires these calls as a further environmental stimulus to reduce and monitor vocal abuse behavior. Program telephone calls require about two minutes per day of the clinician's time.

Reinforcements. Two types of reinforcements are used in the VARP: small weekly reinforcements for bringing in the data consistently, and

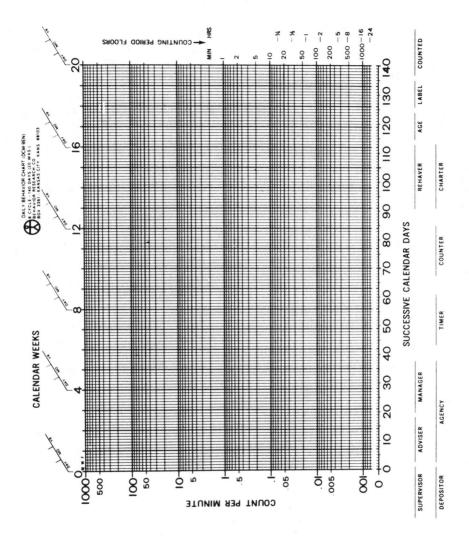

A

Figure 1. *A*, The VARP is most effective when the standard Daily Behavior Chart is used. One advantage to this chart is its capability of demonstrating visually the client's progress through the time being monitored. Keeping accurate data, such as shown in *B*, is also helpful when clinicians need to summarize data for reports presentations and so forth.

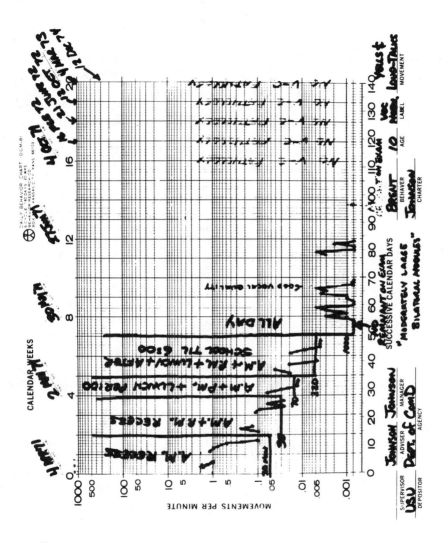

Figure 1,B. See legend on preceding page.

a substantial final reinforcement agreed upon under contract by the parents, the child, and the clinician. (Adults in the program will probably not need external tangible reinforcers as their reinforcers will likely be more intrinsic.)

The small weekly reinforcement is given contingent on consistent and complete data collection by the client. It is not contingent on the frequency of vocal abuse behavior, because low counts may be reported if the reinforcer were contingent upon such performance. Hence, this reinforcer is simply designed to reinforce the child's keeping and bringing in his or her complete weekly record. The small reinforcer also provides a tangible positive result for the child's efforts rather than relying wholly on the final reinforcer which is a distant goal early in the program.

The final reinforcer is the most important one for it supplies the incentive for the client to work toward the goal of remediation of his or her laryngeal problem. The reinforcer is given only when the laryngeal pathology is no longer observed by the physician or laryngologist who originally diagnosed the structural problem. The final reinforcer is agreed to by the child and his or her parents, and a contract is written, signed by the client, his parents, the clinician, and is then notarized by a notary public or initialed by the school principal (notarizing adds a bit of legal flavor to the contract and is of some motivational value). The client is then given one copy of the contract and the clinician keeps the other on file. (See Figure 2 for a sample contract.) The final reinforcer should be something of sufficient value to the client that he will indeed work hard to get it, otherwise he or she may not be motivated to continue in the program. Additionally, the client and parents must understand that the client will not receive the reinforcer until the physician or laryngologist certifies that the larynx has cleared (nodules or polyps gone, thickened cords normal, and so forth). In a pilot study of this program, a six year old girl was working for a bicycle as her final reinforcer. After four weeks of therapy, an increase in vocal abuse was noted as well as a lack of interest in the therapy process. In trying to detect the cause for the increase, it was discovered that the girl had already been able to ride her bicycle as the parents had already purchased it. When asked why she had received her bicycle before her vocal nodules were gone, she replied: "Oh! I don't get the bike until they are gone, but I can ride it if I ask." The program was unsuccessful in controlling her behavior because the power of the reinforcer was for all practical purposes gone. Hence, it is extremely important that everyone understand completely that the reinforcer is neither purchased nor available to the child unless the laryngeal problem is resolved. (Final

CONTRACT AGREEMENT

THIS AGREEMENT made in triplicate this_____day of_____in the year of our
Lord nineteen hundred eighty-____by and between _____,
hereinafter to be referred to as the client, and _____,
hereinafter to be referred to as the parent, is hereby witnessed by_____,
hereinafter to be referred to as the clinician. This conrast shall be held in the files of the clinician until all parts are fulfilled in full to the satisfaction of the said clinician.

THE CLIENT DOES HEREBY AGREE TO :

1. Attend therapy sessions.
2. Supply weekly data, as requested by the speech clinician.
3. Receive the final reinforcement, as stated below, only if, and when _____
   are eliminated as reported by the laryngologist.

THE PARENT DOES HEREBY AGREE TO:

1. Furnish the final reinforcement, as stated below, upon completion of this
   contract by the client.
2. Never allow the client the use or possession of the said final reinforcement
   until the client's___ _____ are eliminated as reported by the
   laryngologist.

FINAL REINFORCEMENT:

The final reinforcement for successful completion of this therapy program (that is, the
elimination of the client's_____as reported by the laryngologist), as agreed
upon jointly by the client and parent shall be:

_____

EXECUTED IN TRIPLICATE THE DAY AND YEAR FIRST ABOVE WRITTEN

_____
(signature of client)

_____
(signature of parent)

_____
(signature of clinician)   WITNESSED

Figure 2. Contract Agreement: This form is used in conjunction with the outlined VARP
steps. This contract is agreed to during the first VARP therapy session with the parent
present. The contents of the contract are self-explanatory. It should be noted, however,
that the final reinforcement is contingent upon vocal pathology being eliminated *as reported
by the physician*. During the Montana VARP Research project, final reinforcements ran
the gamut from a football helmet, a trip to the Dairy Queen, and G.I. Joe clothes, to roller
skates, and a clock radio.

reinforcers have ranged in value from $0.79 model airplanes or games to $80 bicycles. Most children on the program have chosen very frugal reinforcers rather than expensive ones.)

Social reinforcement in the form of encouragement and praise for progress should be given frequently during the course of the program. The clinician may also reinforce the program by finding creative ways for making the sequence fun, thus keeping the client's motivation high.

Awareness Practice. VARP utilizes a procedure for having the client demonstrate various vocal abuse behaviors in order to give him or her an auditory-kinesthetic awareness as to what the abuse behavior sounds and feels like. This increases the client's accuracy at identifying and tallying vocal abuse behaviors which are pinpointed by the clinician as being important and worthy to reduce. The procedure also allows the clinician to teach the client his perception of what should be included within the broad range of the vocal abuse behavior being considered. It is important, for example, for the client to know the difference between loud talk and normal talk. The client needs to hear the difference, feel the difference, and know what it is that the clinician means by loud talking and normal talking. This training is important in the therapy sequence as is demonstrated by the following example: An 11 year old boy was assigned to count loud talks and yells as his pinpointed vocal abuse behavior. At the end of the week, he had counted only 11 instances of loud talks and yells during the entire week. This was unlikely to be sufficient abuse to have caused his vocal nodules. He was given awareness practice training during the session and the next week he returned having monitored 80 loud talks and yells per day. Hence, awareness practice training was found to be an essential part of the VARP procedure. Additionally, overcounting would seem to be better than undercounting.

Initial Session—Parental Involvement. The initial therapy session is a lengthy but necessary session for beginning the VARP. Case history data should be obtained at this time with specific reference to investigating the client's vocal abuse behaviors and the types of high probability situations in which they occur. This is the most efficient time to find out these critical bits of information with the parent or parents and the client present. In addition, many parents and children do not know what the laryngeal pathology really is or what it means even after they have been to the physician or laryngologist. Many fears and anxieties may be relieved through a thorough and sensitive discussion of the problem with both the parents and the child or the adult voice client. This initial session also provides a setting where the final reinforcer contract may be written and agreed upon following an explanation of the therapy process and procedures.

The VARP is a most effective program with good parental communication and cooperation. A study which looked at the feasibility of reducing parental involvement (Beck, 1974) showed that the efficiency and effectiveness of the program was reduced by 50 to 60 per cent when parent cooperation was not to the standard required by VARP. More recent results (Johnson, 1983) suggest that the program does work effectively in the public school environment without extensive parental involvement. Our current recommendation is to encourage clinicians to foster parental involvement, but to be ready to expect successful results from VARP intervention even without it.

Branching—Clinical Alternatives. There are no formal branching steps or procedures for the VARP due to its peculiar and unique individualized format. However, there are some general considerations if the child is not making progress. These considerations are as follows:

1. Is the individual being run on the VARP as written or on a modification of the program—however small? A modification is not likely to work! Again, everything included in the VARP procedure is there because of repeated experience and/or research results. *Stick to the program!*

2. Is the final reinforcer still powerful or has the client found an alternative to it? A new contract may have to be negotiated and written if the client changes his or her mind about what he or she would like to earn.

3. Are the smaller reinforcers adequate enough to keep the program data coming in?

4. Is therapy fun and reinforcing or is it a "drag"?

5. Have the high probability situations been sequenced appropriately? Do not be in too big of a hurry to get the child counting in a big chunk of time. Returning to an earlier successful stage of the program may be necessary.

6. Has the right pinpoint been found? The history of the development of this program is replete with examples of choosing the wrong vocal abuse pinpoint. Care in the analysis of the environment and in the utilization of the vocal mechanism is imperative to ensure the identification of the major source of abuse or misuse. There is no substitute for careful observation of respiration, resonation, and phonatory behaviors.

7. Can others in the individual's environment be involved in assisting the client to remember his responsibility or to monitor him in addition to his own self-counting? School friends may be implemented to become "voice buddies" or "secret voice agents." Husbands, wives, parents, school teachers, little-league coaches, and so forth, may all be involved in the process if approached correctly. Creativity can be utilized effectively within the context of VARP to reduce abusive vocal behavior.

PROGRAM DANGER SIGNALS

Fortunately, there are some definite signals that become apparent in the VARP procedure which should indicate to the clinician that all is not well. These signals are as follows: missing data in any form is a good indicator that the client is beginning to lose interest and incentive in the program; difficulty in completing telephone contacts with the client; and missed appointments for any reason.

These signals should be responded to immediately. No time should be allowed to pass before attending to these problems. They will not clear themselves up. One should implement the problem solving approach suggested in the *Branching—Clinical Alternatives* section to focus on the probable genesis of the difficulty. Additionally, the clinician should make recommitment contacts with the parents and with the client, and if all else fails, one can use what is called *programmed fear*. This is a last resort measure, however, and the procedure for administering it may be obtained by writing to the author.

TAPE RECORDING

A weekly taped sample of one minute of free conversation and one minute of oral reading of the same material is recommended as an index of vocal quality change during the course of the program. A standardized taping procedure should be used keeping the tape recorder, the settings on the recorder, the room, the microphone placement, distance of the subject from the microphone, and so forth, all constant. This will ensure at least as much as possible that the changes in voice quality are a result of laryngeal change rather than being due to recording differences from time to time. Some clinics have a definite place designed to record high quality tape recordings. Cassette tapes are convenient for use particularly because they are easy to store in files and clinical records. Vocal quality changes may shadow the therapy process in either an immediate or delayed fashion. In about half of hyperfunctional voice patients seen at the USU Speech-Language-Hearing Center further vocal facilitative techniques are needed to achieve good voice quality even after the larynx has returned to a normal condition.

PROGRAM RUN TIME

The initial VARP session requires about one hour with the parents and the child (or with the adult voice client). Subsequent weekly sessions will last approximately 15 minutes. Program run data during the past three years indicated that the program will take from five to 14 weeks to complete, depending on the individual problem. The mean number of weeks from beginning of program to remediation (indicated by indirect laryngoscopy by the physician) has been about nine.

If other voice therapy procedures are to be used in the individual's total therapy program, the time of each session may be extended. It is believed by the author (Johnson, 1974) that in children it is inappropriate to carry on vocal retraining procedures other than VARP until laryngeal remediation has taken place. Once VARP procedures have accomplished the reduction of vocal abuse behavior and the laryngeal structure has returned to normal, then techniques such as those recommended by Boone (1984) may be implemented to improve vocal quality and retrain proper vocal usage.

Chapter 2

Forms and Therapy Materials

SUGGESTED PROGRAM MATERIALS

1. Tape recorder and tape (see section on *Tape Recording*)
2. Wrist counter (Behavior Research Company, Box 3551, Kansas City, KS 66103)
3. Fancy wrist band (optional)
4. Pictures of larynx (additional to those included in program)
5. Pictures of various pathologic conditions of the larynx
6. Daily Behavior Chart (6-cycle) (Behavior Research Company)
7. Index cards for data collection
8. Menu of small individualized reinforcements
9. Therapy contract (see Fig. 2)

PROGRAM ENTRANCE EVALUATION

Two evaluations should be accomplished prior to the initial session of VARP. First, an examination of the laryngeal structure should be completed by a qualified physician or laryngologist. The physician or laryngologist should make a written description of the vocal pathology indicating two parameters: size (small, moderate, large) and position (such as bilateral, or unilateral-left). Therapy should not be instituted with voice cases until laryngeal examination results are known.

The second evaluation should be completed by the speech clinician to establish a baseline of the individual's vocal quality, pitch, loudness, and other parameters of interest. A pure tone hearing test should also be completed in order to rule out potential hearing difficulties. Procedures such as Wilson's voice profiling (Wilson, 1972) and physiological measurements such as those recommended by Beckett (1971) and other voice scientists and as summarized by Johnson (1985) should be considered for use. Boone's (1984) evaluation procedures are useful in initial evaluations of voice problems. Objective phonatory measures are not as yet developed adequately enough to provide definitive assistance to the clinician; however, the technology is developing and it is hoped that eventually phonatory measures may assist the clinician in monitoring the client's remediation progress. Johnson (1985) has suggested a potential battery of such measures for clinical progress evaluation. These measures include the S-Z ratio, phonation time, phonation volume, vital capacity and several other computational measures which provide data sensitive to a laryngeal change.

GENERAL FORMAT INSTRUCTIONS

The VARP format is somewhat different from other programmed approaches to speech and language remediation. The nature of therapy sessions dictated by the VARP did not necessitate the highly structured, behavioral targets and event specification such as those found in other behavioral programs like Gray and Ryan (1973), Mowrer (1971), SWRL (1973), Mowrer, Baker, and Schultz (1970), and Lubbert and colleagues (1972). Therefore, the format and the behavioral objectives of the VARP were arranged in a highly flexible manner. In the initial version of the program (Johnson and Parrish, 1972) the program format was simply a listing of the steps required to run the program. The current version of the program has those steps sequenced more efficiently and has the steps placed under a procedures column with additional evaluation aids listed which the clinician may utilize in assessing the effectiveness of his instructions and the progress of the program. The revised format is designed to be more functional for the clinician, and a new addition is a VARP Progress Summary Sheet which is a check list and log for the clinician to use to monitor progress through the program steps.

The VARP is not intended to be a mechanical cookbook approach to voice therapy, and the clinician should be flexible to his or her own personality and clinical creativity in presenting the structural components of the program. If the basic component procedures are followed rigorously with clinical creativity added by the clinician, the program should progress in an effective and efficient manner.

Data collection is a key element of the program. Daily Behavioral Charts must be kept up-to-date in order to assess whether criterion levels have been met or not. Criterion levels have been specified in the VARP to give the clinician a general guideline for moving from one high probability situation or time period to another. These criterion levels have been determined from the individual data of children who have successfully completed the program with remediation of their laryngeal pathology.

Before entering the program, the activities of the Program Entrance

Evaluation must be completed. Therapy should not be instituted with voice problems of any type until the results of laryngeal examination are known to the clinician.

Additionally, the general voice evaluation including hearing screening should be completed prior to the initial session with the parents and the child (or with the adult client).

CASE MANAGEMENT PROCEDURES FOR VOICE DISORDERS

The following are suggested steps in the management of voice disorders by public school clinicians. This is a checklist of procedures to follow and should be completed essentially in this sequence.

1. Individual is identified (screening, teacher referral) as having a possible voice disorder.

2. Individual is evaluated by the clinician to determine all appropriate dimensions and parameters of vocal production. Use a systematic voice evaluation format.

3. Individual's voice is monitored over a period of four weeks (minimum) to ensure reliability.

4. Obtain tape recorded samples of voice production to document problem. A short standard reading sample is useful.

5. The above information is staffed with another clinician to determine whether a physician referral is appropriate.

6. Schedule a parent conference to gather necessary case history information and acquaint parent with the problem.

7. Facilitate ENT physician examination. Consider the options of individual physician referral or voice clinic. Ensure that physician-clinician and parent communications are established. It is highly desirable for clinician to be present at the time of the ENT examination.

8. Consider justification for managing the individual with a voice disorder. Is it appropriate to proceed with intervention strategies?

9. Appropriate intervention strategies may proceed.

10. Complete post-intervention medical evaluation. Communicate intervention strategies, results and evaluation to ENT physician.

FORMS

The following pages contain samples (not necessarily implied to be examples) of forms used in public school management of voice disorders. Standard formats for gathering observations and histories are important in managing voice disorders. They function as check lists and ensure that all the necessary vocal parameters and history specifically required for voice disorders are gathered.

These forms are not meant to be the definitive ones. If you wish to develop your own form, consult most any textbook in general speech pathology, or textbooks specifically devoted to voice disorders. Some suggested voice evaluation forms can be found in Boone (1980a, 1980b, 1984, Chapter 4), Filter (1982), and Wilson (1979).

Form No. 1. Voice Evaluation and History: This sample two page form was used during the Montana VARP Research project by school clinicians to record basic evaluative and historical information relative to a student's voice disorder. Although more complete information could certainly be obtained, this seemed to be sufficient for the management of these cases. In addition, use of this form provided the clinician with a check list of relevant voice parameters to observe.

Form No. 2, Figures 3 and 4. Physician Laryngeal Evaluation and Diagrams: The sample form of a laryngeal evaluation was used during the Montana Research project. Clinicians were present during the examination (a practice always recommended) to ensure the physician recorded his observations. Some physicians prefer to diagram the vocal pathology. Basic diagrams of the vocal cords and of vocal nodules, as seen in Figures 3 and 4, could be added to this form. Physician evaluation forms should be as simple as possible to facilitate quick and easy use by the physician.

Form No. 3. Physician Referral Form: This form has been used in a school district program for physicians to record observations and examination results. This form is sent either with the parent or in the mail to the physician prior to the examination. The form is *always* accompanied by the clinician's voice evaluation and history (Form No. 1) so the physician has an opportunity to review the clinician's observations. Some physicians prefer an open-ended form such as this to being limited by categories and check lists of other forms.

Form No. 4. Medical History: This form was used during the Montana VARP Research project at the voice clinics to obtain a medical history relating to the voice disorder. Public health nurses interviewed parents to obtain this medical history information, which can also be obtained in conjunction with the voice evaluation process (Form No. 1). This form is useful primarily in conjunction with a large voice clinic, but frequently a nurse in the physician's office will gather similar information from students. It is interesting to note that the items in this medical history were suggested by an ENT physician as being related to these types of pathologic conditions.

Form No. 5. VARP Progress Summary Sheet I: This form is used in conjunction with the outlined VARP program steps on the first and second VARP therapy sessions. The format serves the clinician as a reminder and check list of therapy steps, as well as a log of the first two therapy sessions.

Form No. 6. VARP Progress Summary Sheet II: This form is used in conjunction with the outlined VARP program steps beginning with Session III and continuing to the termination of the program. Again, this format serves the clinician as a reminder and check list of therapy steps as well as a log of therapy sessions throughout the program. One of these forms is completed by the clinician during each therapy session.

FORM #1

VOICE EVAL/HISTORY

NAME: DATE:

ADDRESS: BIRTHDATE:

PHONE: AGE:

SCHOOL: CLINICIAN:

GRADE: TEACHER:

                                               PARENTS:

CLIENT INFORMATION:

1. Description of problem: Hoarse voice quality with phonation breaks; often loses voice before completing sentence/intermittently aphonic.

2. Onset and duration of problem: Mother noted problem in 3rd grade, and he has been more consistently hoarse for the past year and a half. His teachers have noted the problem for the past 2 years.

3. Variation of problem: Hoarseness is more pronounced in the morning and after school. Better on weekends.

4. Description of vocal use: Loud talks, yells and screams are evident while he is participating in sports and while playing at home with his brothers as reported by his mother.

Related

a. surgery: *T. & A. Previously had tubes in both ears.*

b. family speech and voice problems: *none.*

c. previous voice therapy: *none.*

5. General health: *Mother reports general good health with exception of tonsillitis in 1st grade.*

STUDENT AND PARENT OBSERVATIONS: *His mother indicated mild concern, but felt nothing could be done. "I thought he would always talk like that." Mother becomes concerned when he loses his voice. Student does not appear to be concerned, but expressed frustration when he loses his voice. Mother is grateful for possible intervention.*
PHYSICAL MECHANISM:

1. Breath control observed: *shallow breathing*

2. Tension sites observed:

   1. face   *none*
   2. mandible   *none*
   3. neck   *some - infrequent*
   4. general body   *none?*
   5. none

FORM #1 (continued)

3. Other physical observations: *Nothing observable. Mother reported results of physical 2 years ago to be normal. Student wears glasses for astigmatism.*

HEARING

A. Impedance - Tympanogram *Type A Tympanogram in right ear showing normal impedance. Left ear showed Type As indicating possible minimal problems.*

B. Pure tone thresholds

Screened normal at 15 db in right and left except thresholds of 20 db at 500 Hz and 1000 Hz in left.

PHONATION

1. Loudness:

Normal X   Too Loud _____   Too Soft _____   Varies _____

2. Quality:

Breathy _____   Harsh _____   Hoarse X   No Voice _____   Hypernasal _____

Denasal _____   Assimilative Nasality _____   Normal Resonance _____

3. Related Observations:

   Pitch Breaks _____ Phonation Breaks _X_ Hard Glottal Attack _____

   Glottal Fry _____ Spastic Dysphonia _____ Aphonia _____

   Articulation problems _____

4. Pitch Description:

   Ability to discriminate pitch differences ___*Fair*___

   Ability to imitate sequential pitch patterns ___*Poor*___

   Ability to carry a tune ___*Poor — Limited pitch range*___

PHONATION TIME: /a/ is sec. _4_ _4_ _5_ Best _5_

              /s/ in sec. _8_ _10_ _11_ Best _11_

              /z/ in sec. _4_ _7_ _5_ Best _7_

CLINICAL IMPRESSIONS OF STUDENT:

Student lacks understanding of problem at this point. Teacher indicates he is above average student and easy to motivate.

_____
Examiner

FORM #2

PHYSICIAN LARYNGEAL EVALUATION

NAME _____   DATE OF EXAMINATION _____

ADDRESS _____   PRE/DURING/POST _____

PHONE _____   BIRTHDATE _____

SCHOOL _____   AGE _____

TEACHER _____ _____   CLINICIAN _____

GRADE _____

1. Statement of condition of laryngeal mechanism (Nodule, Polyp, Thickened Cord, etc.)

vocal cord nodules

2. Statement of size and extent (Large, Moderately Large, Small)

moderate in size

3. Statement of the site of the pathology (Unilateral, Bilateral, Anterior 1/3 or cord, etc.).

ant. 1/3 of each cord

_____
Physician Signature

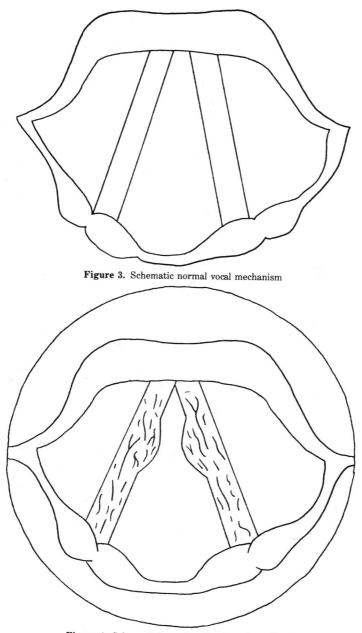

Figure 3. Schematic normal vocal mechanism

Figure 4. Schematic hyperfunctional vocal mechanism
(vocal nodules, nodes, polyps, thickened cords, etc.)

FORM #3

Great Falls Public Schools
Great Falls, Montana
SPEECH AND HEARING SERVICES

Physician Referral Form

STUDENT _____ B/D _____ AGE _____ GRADE _____

SCHOOL _____ DATE OF REFERRAL _____

TO PHYSICIAN: The above student has been asked to consult you because of an
identified communication problem. It would be helpful for our
case management procedures to have a medical description of the
problem. Please review the attached client information data
which describes the observable characteristics of this problem.

PHYSICIAN'S EXAMINATION AND DESCRIPTION OF PROBLEM:

If follow-up examination is indicated, please specify.

Return this report to:
SPEECH AND HEARING SERVICES
Special Education Center
801 Second Avenue North
Great Falls, Montana 59401

Signature of Physician

Address

Date of Examination

FORM #4

MONTANA VARP PROJECT

Medical History

NAME _____   DATE _____

1. History of bacterial infection (tonsils, adenoids, sinus infection).

    T & A 1971. History of frequent tonsillitis and sore
    throats. Surgery by Dr. _____

2. History of virus infection (colds, flu).

    Frequent colds and upper respiratory until after T & A.

3. History of allergy (hayfever, asthma, hives, eczema, food allergy, molds).

    Negative

4. History of exposure to irritants (natural gas, automobile exhaust, tobacco smoke).

Father chain smoker. Cigarette smoke prominent in home.

5. History of trauma to larynx (being choked or strangled, severe blows to neck, inhalation of hot fumes, inhalation of caustic or acid fumes).

Negative

6. History of metabolic imbalance.

7. History of neurologic disturbances.

Concussion Feb. 1974. Treated by neurosurgeon. Fell from bike, injured back of head. Headaches following injury. None now except after playing hard.

FORM #5

VARP PROGRESS SUMMARY SHEET I

(Sessions I and II)

Client _____   Entrance Date _____

Laryngeal Examination Results: *Moderately large nodules on ant. 1/3 of cords.*

Voice Evaluation Findings: *Hoarse; phonation breaks; intermittently aphonic.*

Do not proceed until the Program Entrance Evaluation Results are received.

SESSION I   Completed   Not Completed

1. Case History . . . .   ✓   _____

2. Explanation of the Larynx, etc. . . .   ✓   _____

                    I   Step 4

   2A Normal Larynx   ✓✓   ✓
   2B Superior View   ✓✓   ✓✓
   2C Pathology Picture   ✓✓   ✓✓
   2D Vocal Consequences   ✓✓   ✓

3. Explanation of the therapy program . . . . . .

       I   Step 5

   3A   Goal of Program
   3B   Self-Counting
   3C   Daily Behavior Chart
   3D   Telephone Calls
   3E   Reinforcements
   3F   Parental Involvement

4. Explanation of Larynx to Client . . . .

   4A   Repeating steps

5. Explanation of the therapy program to client .

   5A   Repeating steps

   Comments:

6. Teach Wrist Counter Behavior . . . .

7. Teach 3 x 5 Card Recording . . . .

8. Set up Telephone time . . . .

   Record time: 6:30 P.m.

Form 5 (*continued*).

	Completed	Not Completed
9. Identify forms of vocal abuse	✓	___
Describe: *yells, screams, loud talks*		
10. Identify high probability situations or times . .	✓	___
10A Determine which situations	✓	
10B Rank the situations		
Describe: (1) *after school (3:30 – 5:00) participating in sports.* (2) *A.M. recess* (3) *P.M. Recess or gym* (4) *lunch recess* (5) *8:00 - 8:30 A.M. (Bus stop)* (6) *6:30 – 8:30 (with brothers at home)*		
11. Teach Discrimination of Vocal Abuse	✓	___
12. Determine initial high probability situations . .	✓	___
Describe:		
12A Wearing instructions for WC	✓	
Remind of card recording		
13. Tape recording	✓	___
14. Complete Reinforcement Contract		___
(May be delayed until Session II)		
✓ Delayed to Session II		

15. Set up regular weekly appointment time . . . . . . | ✓

Appointment time:

Wednesday 2:00 - 2:15

SESSION II

1. Collect data and reinforce if appropriate . . . | ✓

2. Review pinpoint and discrimination tasks. . . . | ✓

3. Assigned times for monitoring communicated . . . | ✓

Describe: *Added 15 minutes (P.M. Recess)*

4. Tape recording . . . . | ✓

5. Chart the data . . . . | ✓

6. Rearrange phone and appointment . . . . . . | ✓

Describe: *Continue same time every other night*

7. Contract completed . . . . | ✓

Reinforcement - football helmet with built-in radio

FORM #6

VARP PROGRESS SUMMARY SHEET II

(Sessions III - Termination)

Client _____

Entrance Date _____

Session Number   *3*

Step	Completed	Not Completed
1. Collect, Review and Chart the Data	✓	
Comments:		
2. Review pinpoint, do discrimination-negative practice	✓	
Comments:		
3. Assigned times for monitoring arranged	✓	
Describe assigned times: *Added A. M. Recess*		
4. Tape recording (standard procedure)	✓	

5. Rearrange phone and appointment times . . . . . . /

 Describe times (phone): *Same*

 (appointment):

6. Phonation time: /a/ in sec. 5 4 6 Best 6

7. /s/ in sec. 9 9 10 Best 10

8. /z/ in sec. 4 8 6 Best 8

SESSION COMMENTS: Describe branching, facilitative techniques, other therapy approaches used, problems noted, important parent or client observations, etc.

Student was limiting activities during his count time in order to reduce counts. I called his mother and discussed this with student. He seemed to understand. I had to re-instruct him regarding data card.

_____
Clinician's signature

_____
Session date

Chapter 3

Program Procedures

VOCAL ABUSE REDUCTION PROGRAM
Session I

STEP	PROCEDURES	EVALUATION AIDS
1	Clinician takes case history from parent or parents.	Was information found about high probability situations and the types of vocal abuse behaviors in the child's behavior?
2	Clinician explains the larynx, vocal cords and the laryngeal pathology presented to the parents.	Parents should indicate understanding before proceeding to next step.
2A	Show the pictures of normal larynx. Make the following points: a. larynx often referred to as voice box. b. made of muscle and cartilage. c. vocal folds or cords are muscles. d. vocal cords vibrate when sound is made.	
2B	Show picture of superior view of cords. a. demonstrate how they open and close. b. indicate when child abuses the voice how the cords close together with increased force. c. if it persists a redness or swelling may occur and the cords may become hardened like a callus.	Ask parents if they understand and if they have any questions about the process.

d. describe relationship with their child's diagnosed problem (nodules, polyps, etc.).

e. gets progressively larger and interferes with the vibration of the cords and so the voice is hoarse or breathy.

Ask the parents if there is anything about this which they do not completely understand.

2C Show picture of pathology appropriate to the diagnosed problem (nodules, polyps, etc.)

a. again, describe abuse process and its resultant effect on the voice.

2D Describe to the parents the consequences of the laryngeal pathology remaining.

a. child can't use voice correctly.

b. chances for good voice quality reduced.

c. if pathologic condition becomes too large then it may have to be surgically removed.

3 Clinician explains the therapy program to the parent.

Ask the parents if any of these reasons indicate a need for voice therapy and if they are of sufficient importance to merit cooperation and work. (Note: A negative response here may indicate that they in fact do not see the need or that they cannot get involved in the process. Probe deeper.)

3A Explain that the goal of the program is to reduce the amount of vocal abuse the child is doing during the day.

a. abuse is the cause of the problem.

b. if it is reduced, the problem will diminish.

Ask the parents if they believe that their child is abusing his or her voice and if so how frequently and where. Find out whether they believe that it is possible to eliminate or reduce that abuse.

Session I

STEP	PROCEDURES	EVALUATION AIDS
3B	Explain the self-counting.	
	a. show the wrist counter and demonstrate how it should be worn and how to tally vocal abuses when they occur.	
	b. it is like a string around the finger and it makes the child or client more aware.	
	c. only small periods of time will be counted at first, but eventually the client or child will be responsible for counting the whole day.	Ask the parents if they believe that their child would be able to do such a task. Answer any concern that may be expressed about distraction in school, etc.
	d. the client will keep his or her data for each day on a 3 by 5 inch card (show) which he or she will have to bring to therapy every week. If it is not brought, the client cannot get in. It is like a ticket for entrance.	
	e. Describe the content on the card (date, count, and time counted).	
3C	Show the Daily Behavior Chart.	Ask the parents whether the child will do this faithfully.
	a. explain that you will keep the client's count data on the chart to assess progress.	
	b. goal is to reduce the frequency or to make the line on the chart go down.	

3D Explain the weekly sessions.

a. once a week for about 15 minutes.

b. activities will be: taping, charting data, instructions for the next week, and encouragement to keep trying.

Ask the parents if that schedule will be convenient and possible for them.

3E Explain the telephone calls.

a. every day for first two weeks to obtain daily data and to act as a reminder.

b. as the client progresses in the program there will be fewer calls.

c. eventually calls will not be necessary.

Ask the parents their opinion on the best time each day to call and catch the child at home.

3F Explain the reinforcements.

a. small reinforcer is given each week when the client brings in data complete. He or she will choose it from a variety of things.

b. show contract. As an incentive for getting rid of his vocal problem, we will contract with you and the child for him to receive something he has wanted very much. When the doctor says the problem is resolved then the item may be purchased for the child. Not before (be sure to stress the contingency part).

Ask the parents if they will agree to the contract with their child on this basis.

Session I

STEP	PROCEDURES	EVALUATION AIDS
	c. must not receive the item until the doctor has indicated that the problem with the larynx is resolved.	Ask the parents if they understand the terms of the program and if they are willing to assist in this way.
3G	Explain how they (parents) can help.	Ask the parents if there are any further questions regarding the problem or the therapy.
	a. furnishing the final reinforcer and keeping the contract.	
	b. make sure the wrist counter goes with the child when necessary.	
	c. make sure the child makes his telephone contacts with the clinician.	
	d. see that the child gets to his weekly appointments and arrange for cancellations if necessary.	
	e. be a general monitor as to how the child is progressing.	
4	Child is given explanation of the larynx, vocal cords and the laryngeal pathology which he or she has.	

4A	Repeat Steps 2A, 2B, 2C, 2D.	Ask the child questions which will probe his or her understanding of the general problem.
5	Client is given an explanation of the therapy program.	
5A	Repeat Steps 3A, 3B, 3C, 3D, 3E, 3F.	Ask the child periodic questions that will probe his or her understanding of the therapy program and goals. Get a general subjective reaction to whether or not the child will cooperate and do the necessary work.
6	Teach the client wrist counter behavior. a. tally using the response plunger. b. resetting to zero using the dials on the face.	Have the child tally up to 12. Have him or her reset the counter to zero. Repeat, using another higher number.
7	Teach the client how to record on the 3 by 5 inch cards. a. space to record the date. b. space to record number of abuses. c. do it just before going to bed.	Have him or her fill in a card with some theoretical data and check the work. Ask the child if he or she understands everything so far.

Session I

STEP	PROCEDURES	EVALUATION AIDS
8	Set up desirable telephone call time.	Have him or her write the agreed upon time on a 3 by 5 card to be placed in his or her room.
	Find out what would be a convenient time to call. Tell him what you will want to know when you call.	
	a. any problems with counting. b. how many counted today.	
9	Find out from the client what kinds of vocal abuse behaviors he does frequently.	
9A	Vocal abuse is defined in terms of the individual client. Find out which vocal abuses occur most frequently in his opinion. The following is a list of possible abusive behaviors:	Ask the client if he or she ever thought that these things were hard on the voice box.
	loud talking yelling throat clearing coughs motor noises (during play) shouting	Determine how the client feels about trying to change some of these abuses and if he or she thinks it is possible to change.

crying
singing

This step is very closely related to step 10 so overlap of information is to be expected in these two steps.

10   Identify from the client's environment (by interview) situations where a high probability for vocal abuse exists.

10A   From the list of high probability situations determine which are appropriate to the client. In addition, ask the client if there are other situations in which he uses his voice a lot. When a relevant list has been compiled rank them from most frequent to least frequently occurring situations.

    recesses
    lunch break
    music class
    little league
    swimming
    gym class
    cub scouts
    after school
    home activities
    bike riding
    weekend activities

Session I

STEP	PROCEDURES	EVALUATION AIDS
11	Teach the client to beware of his own vocal abuse behavior. Explain how to distinguish between, for example, loud talking and normal talking if loud talking has been pinpointed as a primary abuse pinpoint.	Probe to find out whether the client knows what is meant by the vocal abuse pinpoints identified in Step 9A.
11A	Do any *two* of the following three procedures: a. The client will talk in a normal voice and then in a loud voice and record them on several separate Language Master cards. Mix the cards and have the client identify the loud talking ones. b. Role play different situations, having the client count on the wrist counter when he emits a vocal abuse pinpoint. c. Use a tape recorder with a VU meter. Tape the client, having him voluntarily peak the needle several times. Play the tape back and have him watch and listen for the abuses.	Performance on discrimination of those tasks.

12	Decide with the client on the first short high probability situation during which the client will be counting his pinpointed vocal abuses during the next week.	Have the client write this on the 3 by 5 index card as a reminder.
12A	Instruct him to wear his wrist counter only during the selected time. He is not to wear it at other times during the day. He must carry it in the pocket during the remainder of the day. Remind him to record the day's tally in the appropriate space on the index card before going to bed.	Have the child write that on the card as well.
13	Tape record one minute sample of conversation and oral reading (use a standard reading passage). (Use standardized recording techniques—see section on tape recording.)	
14	Bring parents back into the session and complete the final reinforcer contract if possible before terminating the session. If a decision cannot be reached, the client may take the contracts with him to be agreed upon and signed at home. He must return them, however, by the next therapy session.	
15	Set up regular weekly appointment time for the client.	

Session II

STEP	PROCEDURES	EVALUATION AIDS
1	Collect the data for the week and review the client's reactions and problems if any.	
1A	If the data are complete and appropriately recorded, administer the small reinforcer.	
2	Review the pinpointed abusive vocal behavior and do some discrimination negative practice tasks as described in Session I Step 11A. (Creative procedures by individual clinicians would be appropriate here.)	Monitor whether the client seems to be able to discriminate the vocal abuse and if he or she is comfortable in counting it.
3	Instruct the client to continue monitoring the pinpointed behavior in the same high probability situation for another week.	Have the child write it down again on another index card.
4	Tape record one minute sample of conversation and oral reading using the same standardized procedure as described previously.	
5	Chart the collected data on the Daily Behavior Chart and show to the client.	

STEP	PROCEDURES	EVALUATION AIDS
6	Rearrange the telephone call contact times and reconfirm the next clinical appointment.	Have him or her write it on the index card.

Session III

STEP	PROCEDURES	EVALUATION AIDS
1	Collect the data for the week and review with the client. Chart the data on the Daily Behavior Chart.	
1A	If the data are complete, give an appropriate reinforcer.	
2	Review the pinpointed abusive vocal behavior and do some discrimination negative practice tasks.	
3	According to the data, extend the self-counting to a second time period or situation if the client demonstrated the establishment of control over the vocal abuse pinpoint during the initial two weeks. Criterion for moving on: one to two vocal abuse pinpoints during the last two days.)	Client must have met criterion before additional time or situations are added. Have him or her write the new situation on an index card and include the older situation as well.
4	Tape record one minute sample of conversation and oral reading using the same standardized procedure as described previously.	

Session III

STEP	PROCEDURES	EVALUATION AIDS
5	Give the client a new index data collection card.	
6	Rearrange the telephone call contact times and reconfirm the next clinical appointment.	Have the client write it on the instruction card.

Session IV

STEP	PROCEDURES	EVALUATION AIDS
1	Collect and chart the data for the week and review with the client.	(Criterion for moving on: one to two vocal abuse behaviors during the final two days of the reported week.)
1A	If the data are complete, give the reinforcer.	
2	Review the pinpointed abusive vocal behavior and do some discrimination negative practice tasks.	

3   According to the data, extend the self-counting to an additional time period or situation. If the client did not meet the criterion level one to two vocal abuse behaviors during the final two days of the week), then or she should continue with the situation or time period of the previous week.   Have him or her write any changes on the instruction card.

4   Tape record one minute sample of conversation and oral reading using the standardized taping procedure.

5   Rearrange the telephone contact times to occur only two to three times per week (as needed).   Have the client write this change on the instruction card.

6   Reconfirm the next clinical appointment.

Session V

STEP	PROCEDURES	EVALUATION AIDS
1	Collect, chart, and review the data with the client.	(Criterion for moving on: one to two vocal abuses during the final two days of the reported week.)
1A	If the data are complete, give the reinforcer.	
2	Review the pinpointed abusive vocal behavior and do some discrimination negative practice tasks.	
3	If appropriate according to the data, extend the self-counting to an additional time period or situation. *Note criterion level.*	Have the client write any changes on his or her instruction card.
	If criterion was not met continue working on the situation or time period used during the previous week.	
4	Tape record one minute sample of conversation and oral reading using the standardized taping procedure.	
5	Rearrange the telephone contact times to occur only one to two times per week (as needed).	Have the client write this change on his or her instruction card.
6	Reconfirm the next clinical appointment.	

Session VI and all subsequent sessions

STEP	PROCEDURES	EVALUATION AIDS
1	Collect, chart, and review the data with the client.	(Criterion for moving on: one to four vocal abuses during the final two days of the reported week.)
1A	If the data are complete, give the reinforcer.	
2	Review the pinpointed abusive vocal behavior and do some discrimination negative practice tasks.	
3	If appropriate according to the data, extend the self-counting to an additional time period or situation. *Note criterion level.*	
	If criterion was not met, continue working on the situation or time period used during the previous week.	Have the client write any changes on the instruction card.
4	Tape record one minute sample of conversation and oral reading using the standardized taping procedure.	
5	Rearrange the telephone contact times to occur only once a week or eliminate them (as necessary).	Have the client write any changes on the instruction card.
6	Reconfirm the next clinical appointment.	

Note:
Sometime between the sixth and eighth weeks, an appointment should be made with the original physician or laryngologist by the parents to examine the laryngeal structure. Laryngeal changes should be apparent by this time if the program is running properly. If little or no structural change is noted, then pinpoints should be carefully analyzed and the validity of the data must be looked at carefully. Clients running on the VARP procedure should be seen minimally every three months for indirect laryngoscopy.

Additional program sessions. The remainder of the VARP will follow the previous session outlines until the client is counting all day or until the laryngeal pathology is eliminated. If the all-day goal is reached and on examination the laryngeal pathology is still present, a program allowing a maximum of two vocal abuses per day should be followed until the pathology is eliminated. A periodic recheck every two to six months should be conducted by the laryngologist. Discrimination negative practice tasks may be eliminated in the subsequent sessions unless new vocal abuse behaviors are pinpointed.

REFERENCES

Beck, M. (1974). *The remediation of vocal nodules in school children: A therapeutic program.* Unpublished master's thesis, Utah State University, Logan.

Beckett, R. L. (1971). The respirometer as a diagnostic and clinical tool in the speech clinic. *Journal of Speech and Hearing Disorders, 37*(2), 235–241.

Boone, D. R. (1980a). *The Boone voice program for children.* Austin, TX: PRO-ED.

Boone, D. R. (1980b). *The Boone voice program for adults.* Austin, TX: PRO-ED.

Boone, D. R. (1984). *The voice and voice therapy* (3rd ed.) Englewood Cliffs, NJ: Prentice-Hall.

Bryce, D. P. *Differential diagnosis and treatment of hoarseness.* Springfield, IL: Charles C Thomas.

DeWeese, D. D., and Saunders, W. H. (1973). *Textbook of otolaryngolology.* St. Louis: C. V. Mosby.

Diedrich, W. M. (1974). *Charting speech behavior.* Lawrence, KS: University of Kansas, Extramural Independent Study Center.

Edwards, K. A., and Powers, R. B. (Eds.) (1973). *Self control: Contemporary approaches with a behavioral emphasis.* Logan, UT: Utah State University, Department of Psychology.

Foster, C. (1974). *Developing self control.* Kalamazoo, MI: Behaviordelia, Inc.

Gordon, K. (1971). Frustrations of an operant public school therapist dealing with vocal nodules. *Feedback, 5,* 3.

Gray, B. B., and Ryan, B. R. (1973). *A language program for the nonlanguage child.* Champaign, IL: Research Press.

Hunsaker, J. C. (1970). *Behavior modification and functional voice disorders.* Unpublished master's thesis, Utah State University, Logan.

Johnson, T. S. (1971). A behavior management approach to vocal nodules in children. *Feedback 3,* 2–3.

Johnson, T. S. (1974, Fall/Winter). A behavioral research approach to the clinical treatment of voice disorders. *Iowa Speech and Hearing Association Journal,* pp. 1–3.

Johnson, T. S. (1983). Treatment of vocal abuse in children. In W. H. Perkins, *Voice disorders.* New York: Thieme Stratton.

Johnson, T. S. (1985). Voice disorders: The measurement of clinical progress. In J. M. Costello (Ed.), *Speech disorders in adults: Recent advances.* San Diego: College-Hill Press.

Johnson, T. S., and Child, D. L. (1984). *VARP: Vocal abuse reduction program— microcomputer program.* Austin, TX: PRO-ED.

Johnson, T. S., and Parrish, M. (1971). A behavior management approach to vocal nodules in children II: Report of cases. *Feedback 4,* 11–12.

Johnson, T. S., and Parrish, M. L. (1972). *A therapeutic program for the systematic remediation of vocal nodules in children.* Logan, UT: Utah State University.

Johnson, T. S., and Wing, D. M. (1976a). *VARP: Precision management of vocal abuse behaviors in children.* Portland, OR: May, 1976, workshop materials, ASHA Western Regional Conference.

Johnson, T. S., and Wing, D. M. (In preparation). Precision management of vocal abuse in children.

Koorland, M. A., and Martin, M. B. (1975). *Elementary principles and procedures of the standard behavior chart.* Gainesville, FL: Learning Environments, Inc.

Kunzelmann, H., Cohen, M. A., Hulten, W. J., Martin, G. L., and Mingo, A. R. (1970). *Precision teaching: An initial training sequence.* Seattle, WA: Special Child Publications.

Lindsley, O. R. (1968). A reliable wrist counter for recording behavior rates. *Journal of Applied Behavior Analysis, 1,* 77.

Lubbert, L. L., Johnson, K., Brenner, C., and Alderson, A. (1972). *Behavior modification articulation program.* Tempe, AR: I.D.E.A.S.

Miller, L. K. (1980). *Principles of everyday behavior analysis.* Monterey, CA: Brooks/Cole Publishing.

Mowrer, D. E. (1971). *Technical Research Report S-1: Reduction of stuttering behavior.* Tempe, AR: Arizona State University Bookstore.

Mowrer, D. E. (1982) *Methods of modifying speech behaviors* (2nd ed.) Columbus, OH: Charles E. Merrill.

Mowrer, D. E., Baker, R. L., and Schultz, R. E. (1970). *Modification of the frontal Lisp-S-Pack.* Palos Verdes Estates, CA: Educational Psychological Research Associates.

Parrish, M. L. (1972). *A therapeutic program for the remediation of vocal nodules in children.* Unpublished master's thesis, Utah State University, Logan.

SWRL (1973). *SWRL articulation programs.* New York: Southwestern Regional Laboratory—American Book Company.

Thompson, C. (1976). *The feasibility of using respirometer measurements as a monitoring agent of laryngeal functioning during vocal nodule rehabilitation.* Unpublished master's thesis, Utah State University, Logan.

White, O. R., and Haring, N. G. (1980). *Exceptional Teaching.* Columbus, OH: Charles E. Merrill.

Wilson, D. K. (1979). *Voice problems of children.* Baltimore: Williams & Wilkins.

Wilson, F. B. (1972). The voice-disordered child: A descriptive approach. *Language, Speech, and Hearing Services in the Schools, 4,* 14–22.

Wing, D. M., Johnson, T. S., DeVoe, S., and Pearson, M. (1975, September). *Vocal abuse reduction program: A Montana pilot project for the management of children's voice disorders.* Final report, Montana VARP Project, Montana Office of the Superintendent of Public Instruction.

APPENDIX A

Precision Management of Vocal Abuse Behaviors in Children: Workshop Materials

1. Precision Management of Vocal Abuse Behaviors

2. Should we be concerned with hoarseness?

3. Total Impact of Communication =

$$\boxed{7\% \text{ Verbal}} \;+\; \boxed{38\% \text{ Vocal}} \;+\; \boxed{55\% \text{ Facial Visual}}$$

4. Sociological Effects – Psychological Effects – Physiological Effects

5. Potential physiological-medical problems that have persistent hoarseness as one of the symptoms:
   Laryngeal Polyposis, Vocal Nodules, Contact Ulcers, Hyperkeratosis, Leukoplakia, Benign Tumors of the Larynx, Laryngeal Malignancy, Laryngeal Paralysis, Tuberculosis, Syphilis, Juvenile Papillomatosis, Various Types of Laryngitis, Laryngeal Edema, etc.

6. Hoarseness is a symptom that must not be ignored. It is a life threatening symptom. Medical textbooks are very clear as to the importance of this disease symptom (see Brewer attachment):

   DeWeese and Saunders, *Textbook of Otolaryngology*, "Any patient who is hoarse longer than two weeks deserves a careful inspection of the larynx" (p.106).

   Bryce, *Differential Diagnosis and Treatment of Hoarseness*, "Hoarseness which is temporary occurs so commonly that it tends to be disregarded. Unfortunately, very often a more serious disease is misdiagnosed as laryngitis, and thus its diagnosis is delayed. It is essential to realize that hoarseness resulting from acute inflammatory disease of the larynx does not persist, although it may recur. It has been emphasized for many years that the symptom of hoarseness that persists *beyond three weeks* without an accompanying respiratory inflammation must be investigated fully. This can be done by simple, indirect laryngoscopy" (p. 24).

7. Hyperfunction and its Behaviors
   Most voice disorders, 85 to 90 per cent, are related to misuse
   and abuse of the vocal mechanism.

   > Emil Froeschels: "Hyperfunction pertains to all forms of excessive
   > muscular tension in the vocal tract."

   Prolonged hyperfunctional use of the voice exhausts the vocal
   muscles to the degree that they finally become unable to pro-
   duce even a normal degree of tonus and hypofunction sets in.

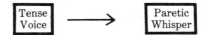

8. The process of hyperfunction that is the mechanism of
   nonmalignant persistent hoarseness includes:

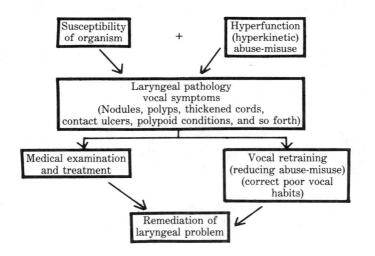

9. Susceptibility factors include:
   (A.) Histologic differences in the basic cellular make-up
   (B.) Presence of an invading organism
   (C.) Vocal conditioning history (analogy with jogging)
   (D.) Other X factors

10. The hyperfunctional equation:

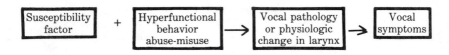

Examples of the hyperfunctional equation:

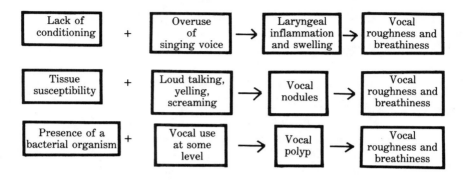

11. Types of hyperfunctional problems:
    (A.) No observable pathology
    (B.) Inflammation–laryngitis
    (C.) Laryngeal polyps
    (D.) Laryngeal polyposis
    (E.) Vocal nodules
    (F.) Contact ulcers

12. Function analysis of voice disorders
    Principle I. Voice and the factors relating to its physiology and pathology are not exempt from the principles of learning. Many voice disorders spring from hyperfunctional action of the structure which can be manipulated behaviorally.
    Principle II. Some voice disorders have primarily an organic basis. The therapeutic techniques used to facilitate a better voice still can take advantage of what we know about the modification of behavior. This fact has been largely neglected in the voice literature.
    Principle III. The utilization of stimulus programming and consequence management should be utilized in voice therapy just as in other areas of speech and language pathology.

13. Treatment model for children with chronic hoarseness resulting from misuse-abuse (hyperfunction)
    (A.) Systematic reduction of vocal misuse-abuse behavior. Much discussion about this—but little in the way of "How does one do it!" Few specific procedures.

(B.) Establishment of good vocal quality.
Most of the discussed therapeutic techniques in the voice literature fall under this category (chewing, pushing, breath control, and so forth).

(C.) Extension—generalization of good vocal quality to all situations.
Little data and or writing in this area.

14. Phonatory hyperfunction occurs at three levels: respiration, phonation, and resonation.
Misuse—Inappropriate physiological functioning of the phonatory systems (Physiological dimension).
Abuse—Straining or excessive use of normal physiology of phonation (psychological or behavioral dimension).

15. Common hyperfunctional behaviors
Respiration
   Speaking on "residual" air or on inhalation
Resonation
   Speaking with taut pharynx
   Speaking with little mouth opening
   Speaking with faulty tongue position
Phonation
   Breathy voice—excessive air flow due to faulty
approximation of vocal cords
   Tight—strained phonation, over-adduction of the vocal cords, hard to get air past the cords
   Hard attack—banging arytenoid cartilages together
   Increasing the loudness of the voice by tension rather than by air
   Loud—talking and yelling
   Cheering, screaming
   Coughing, throat clearing
   Strained vocalizing
   Singing

16. Behavioral control of vocal abuse-misuse
   (A.) Identify hyperfunctional behaviors of importance (misuse-abuse).

(B.) Identify the situations or times during which these have the highest probability of occurring.

(C.) Systematically reduce those behaviors in each situation: Vocal Abuse Reduction Program (VARP)

17. Purpose
    (A.) To pinpoint vocal abuse behavior in individuals with hyperfunctional voice disorders.
    (B.) To systematically reduce the pinpointed vocal abuse behaviors in specific high probability situations.
    (C.) To reduce in size or eliminate laryngeal pathology associated with the hyperfunctional use of the voice—making possible the subsequent establishment of good vocal quality.

18. Program run time
    (A.) Initial session: 30 minutes to 1 hour with client and parents.
    (B.) Subsequent sessions once a week for approximately 15 minutes.
    (C.) Length of program depends on the individual problem. Data indicate range from five to 14 weeks (x = 9.5 weeks)
    (D.) Telephone call time investment: two minutes per day in the early stages, reduced to zero as program progresses.

19. Program components
    (A.) Pinpointing voice abuse-misuse
        •countable and observable
        •individual variations
    (B.) Self-counting
    (C.) Wrist counters (available from Behavior Research Company, PO Box 3351, Kansas City, KS 66103)
    (D.) High probability time periods
        •stimulus control
        •situational control transfer
    (E.) Daily behavior charting
        •standard behavior chart (available from Behavior Research Company)
    (F.) Telephone calls
        •carefully programmed

•faded as program progresses
•necessary for program success
(G.) Reinforcements
•small weekly
•substantial final (contracted)
•contingent

20. Discrimination practice
Auditory—kinesthetic awareness

21. Initial session parental involvement

22. Branching—clinical alternatives
Individualized
Modified VARP or VARP?
Power of reinforcers
Sequencing of steps
Is the pinpoint correct?
Others in the environment as reminder stimuli

23. Vocal abuse pinpoints
Loud talks and yells
Throat clears
Coughs
Hard glottal attacks
Strained vocalizations
Child-play noises
Excessive talking
Crying
Singing
Excessive glottal fry

24. High probability situations and time periods
AM and PM school recesses
Before evening meal
After school before arriving home
Lunch hour
Music class
Bike riding
Little League
Swimming
Cub Scout meetings
Gym class

Home situations

25. Program danger signals
    Missing data in any form
    Difficulty in completing telephone contacts
    Missed appointments
    (*Don't wait around for these to clear themselves up—they won't!*)

26. Suggested solutions and branch steps
    (A.) Check on reinforcers, are they strong and is the terminal one sufficient incentive, and adjust if necessary.
    (B.) "Folks are folks" and "People do well what pays off for them."
    (C.) Parent contact and recommitment.
    (D.) Adjust the program steps to less demanding if necessary; the last jump may be too big.
    (E.) Client discussion and recommitment.
    (F.) Have you run the program as outlined or have you made modifications to it? VARP works! Yours might not.
    (G.) Programmed fear, a last resort.

27. Program supplements
    (A.) Classroom teacher cooperation—inform and involve on limited basis.
    (B.) Peer assistance—a "voice buddy" can remind and watch.
    (C.) Watch the process of voice production carefully and make sure you have the pinpoints identified appropriately. There is no substitute for direct observation. Care enough to observe.

28. Session outline
    (A.) Collect data.
    (B.) Reinforce client for bringing in data.
    (C.) Review the pinpointed abusive vocal behavior and practice vocal discrimination.
    (D.) Instruct client as to pinpointed behavior and high probability situations.
    (E.) Tape record sample of voice.
    (F.) Chart collected data.
    (G.) Rearrange telephone call contact times and confirm next clinical appointment.

29. Program data

	Remedied	Not Remedied	Dropouts
First edition			
1970 (speech clinic)	4	6	3
VNP			
Parrish and Johnson, 1972 (speech clinic)	34	2*	4
Beck School			
Revision, 1973–74 (school district)	3	3†	4
VARP			
1974 (speech clinic)	44	3	5
School District			
1975 (Montana Project)	22‡	2	2

---

* Subsequently remedied on different program
† Includes two children not reexamined by ENT physician
‡ Includes 12 children who had "significant improvement"

APPENDIX B

Case Study—Bret

The following case study report was selected to represent the typical management process of a student in the Montana VARP project.

Bret, age 11, was referred to the speech clinician by his sixth grade teacher because of hoarse voice quality. Bret's mother described his voice as very hoarse and indicated that his hoarseness was more pronounced in the mornings and right after school following periods of yelling. This problem was noted consistently during all speaking situations for the previous year. Bret's hoarseness was accompanied by phonation breaks. Breath control appeared to be normal with no observable tension sites. He was not able to imitate sequential pitch patterns or carry a tune. Other vocal measures and symptoms typified a hyperfunctional voice disorder.

The vocal misuse and abuse behaviors pinpointed were loud talks, frequent yells, and screams while participating in group sports and playing at home with his brother. Bret's mother agreed with these pinpoints and concurred with the identification of the situations. Based on the clinician's voice evaluation and history, Bret was scheduled for a laryngeal examination by an ENT physician during the project voice clinic in Great Falls. Results of this examination revealed the presence of a vocal cord nodule on the anterior one third of the left true cord. Because of his vocal cord pathology, chronic vocal symptoms of hoarseness and a history of vocal abuse–misuse it was decided to place Bret on the VARP. The initial VARP session with Bret, his mother, and the clinician, was scheduled for the following week. During this first 45 minute conference, Bret and his mother became acquainted with the procedures of the VARP and how it might help him reduce or eliminate his vocal nodule. The clinician first explained the larynx, vocal cords and Bret's particular vocal cord pathology (vocal nodule). Vocal abuse behaviors were identified and it was determined that the high probability situations in which they typically occur with Bret were: after school; morning, afternoon, and lunch recesses; early morning before school at the bus stop; and after dinner at home with his brother.

The clinician explained that the goal of the program was to reduce the amount of vocal abuse the child emitted during the day. Bret was given a wrist counter and taught how to count his "yells" at specified high probability times during each day, and record this data on a 3 by 5 inch index card. It was then explained that his daily count data would be transferred to another chart with a goal of reducing the frequency of yells. Bret agreed on a convenient telephone time so that he could be called each night (as per the VARP procedure) by the clinician to discuss any problems and gather his daily count data. Bret, his mother, and the clinician then signed a VARP contract agreement which indicated that if Bret attended weekly therapy sessions and supplied his daily count, he would receive a final reinforcement from his parents only if and when vocal nodules were eliminated as reported by the ENT physician upon final examination. The final reinforcement was agreed upon by Bret and his parents.

Bret began counting his vocal abuse (yells) for 30 minutes each day after school. Within the first week and a half, Bret was able to reduce his vocal abuse from 0.4 yells per minute to 0.0 during this 30 minute period. Afternoon recess was then added for a total of 45 minutes he was responsible to control and count. Bret gradually increased his daily count period until he was able to monitor his vocal behavior for an entire day by the eighth week.

Bret met with his clinician once each week at school for a 15 minute therapy session. During this time, his data was collected and recorded on the chart, vocal abuse behaviors were reviewed, counting times were assigned, a voice sample was recorded, and other phonation measures were sampled. Additionally, Bret and the clinician solved problems as they arose during the course of the program according to the problem solving guide in the VARP manual.

At the end of 16 weeks, Bret returned to the ENT physician for a post-intervention examination of the larynx. Results of that examination indicated that the vocal nodule had reduced significantly in size such that only a tiny remnant of the former nodule could be seen.

Bret's chart (see Figure 5) shows the deceleration of vocal abuse behavior over the course of 16 weeks (116 days). His initial rates of vocal abuse behavior were about 0.4 per minute on the chart, which translates to 12 yells in the 30 minutes he initially began counting. By the fifth day of his counting, Bret had reduced his vocal abuse behaviors to zero in the 30 minute period of time he was monitoring (zero is charted beneath the 30 minute "floor" line drawn horizontally on the chart for the first nine days of the chart). By gradually increasing the amount of time he is responsible for and by Bret's reducing abuse-misuse in a like manner during those periods, he was able to progress to counting all day by the middle of the ninth week. At that point Bret was having four to ten vocal abuse behaviors during the entire day, and he reduced that to one or two and finally to zero by the fourteenth to fifteenth week. Computing the acceleration of the data (Koorland and Martin, 1975) reveals that Bret's deceleration was $\div 1.5$ (divide by 1.5, indicating a 50 per cent decrease per week in vocal abuse–misuse behavior).

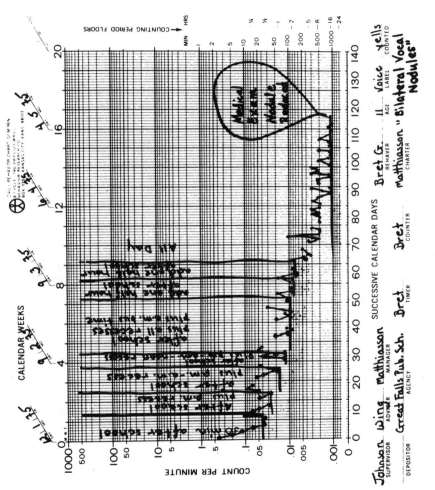

Figure 5